THE MINDFUL FENNEC FOX

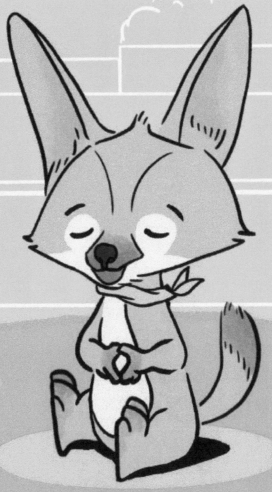

A CHILDREN'S BOOK ABOUT PATIENCE, SLOWING DOWN, AND BALANCE

WRITTEN BY
CHARLOTTE DANE

ILLUSTRATED BY
ADAM RIONG

THE MINDFUL FENNEC FOX

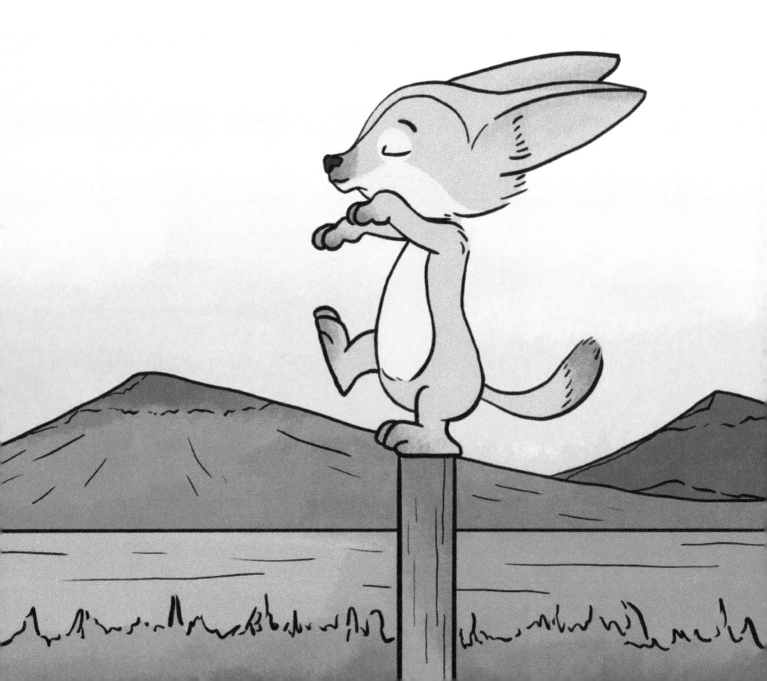

Fennec Fox was well-known for being able to remain calm under pressure. His emotions never controlled or distracted him.

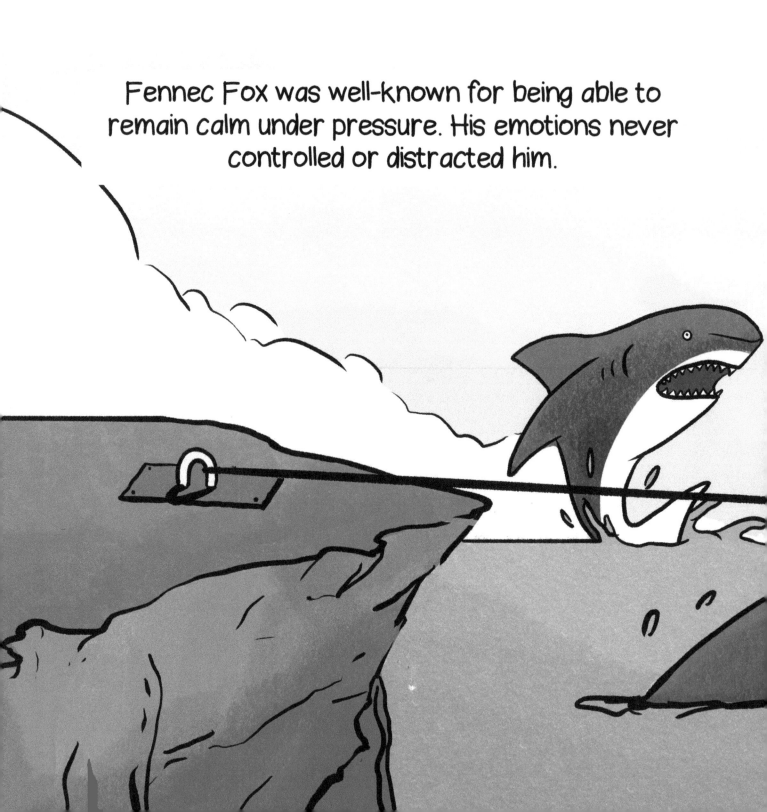

Our brains can be very noisy, and Fennec Fox could tune everything out to relax and focus.

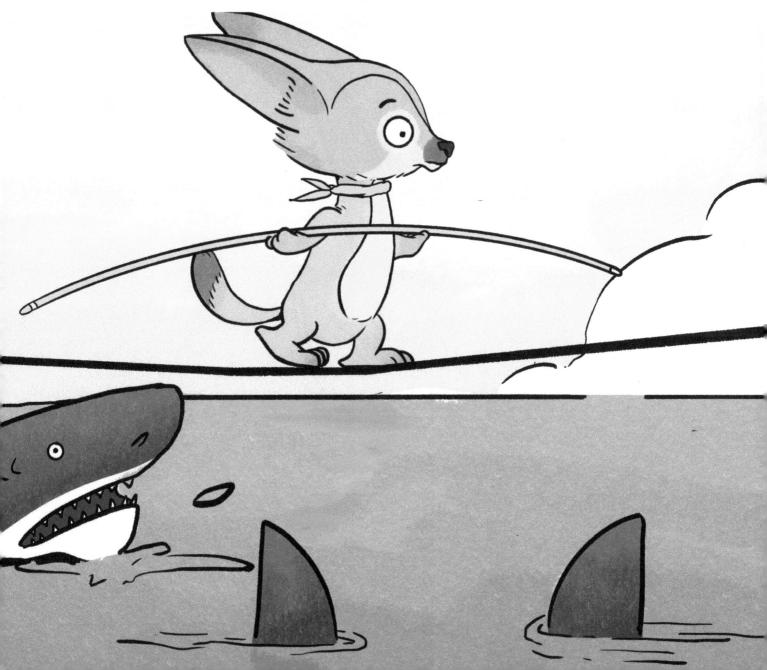

Of course he worried and overthought things like many of his friends, but he would always manage to excel at the task at hand.

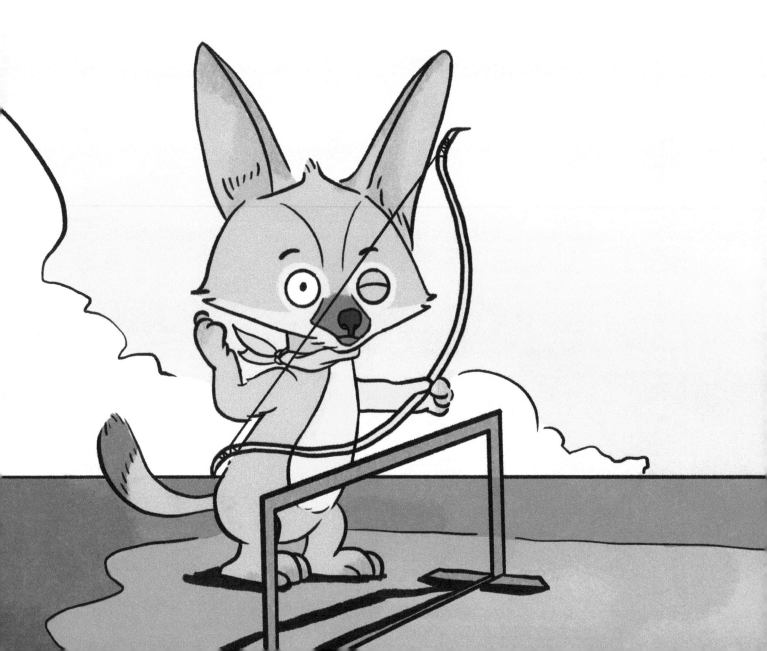

He was so mindful that he didn't even have to try anymore.

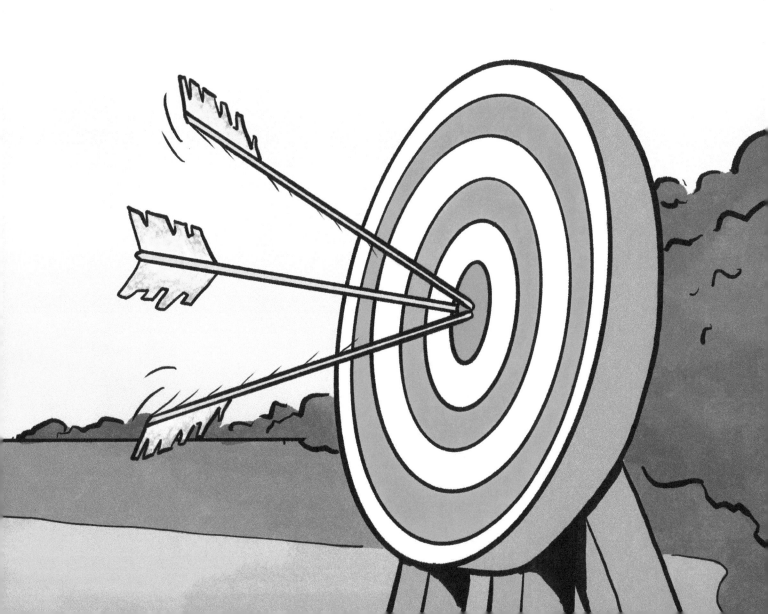

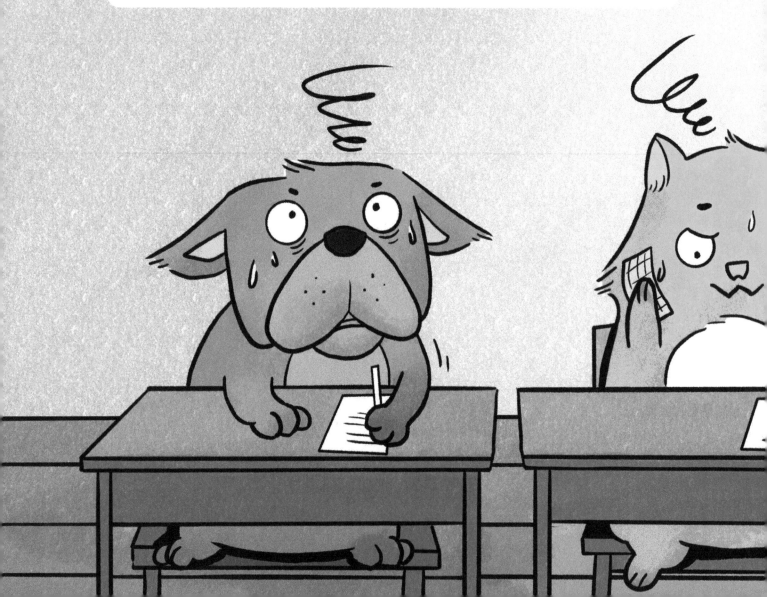

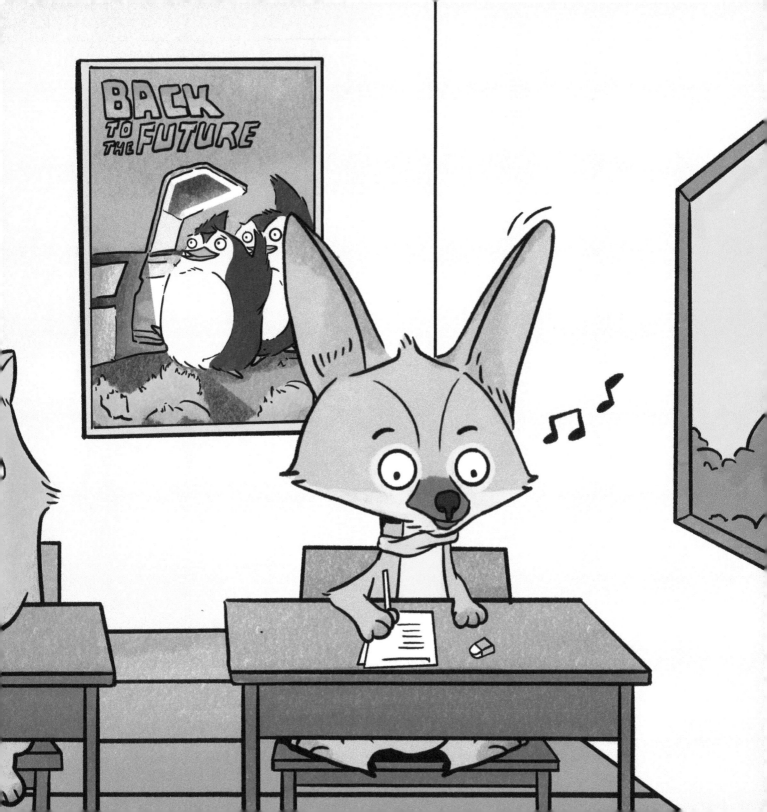

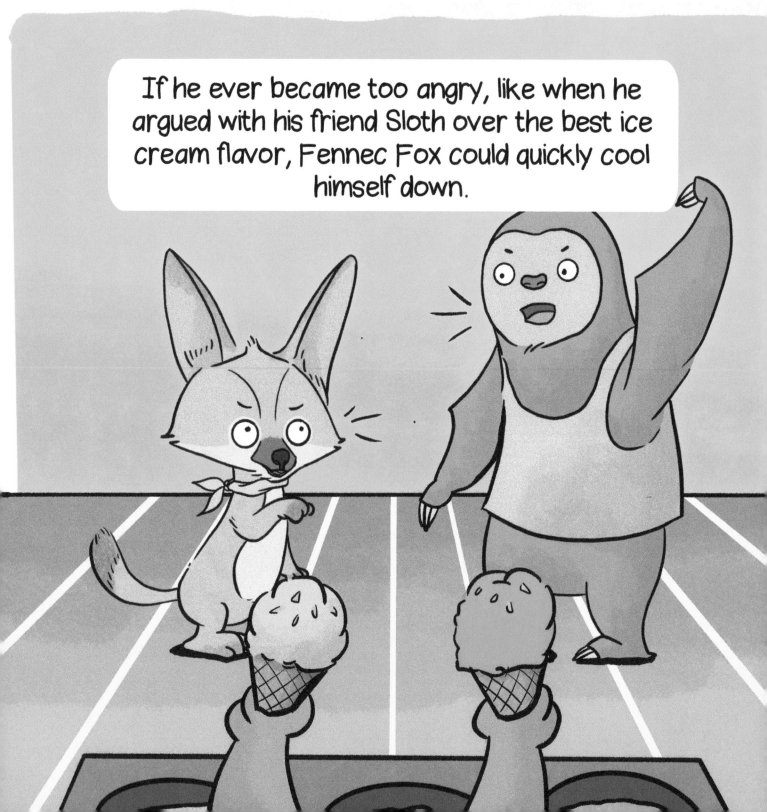

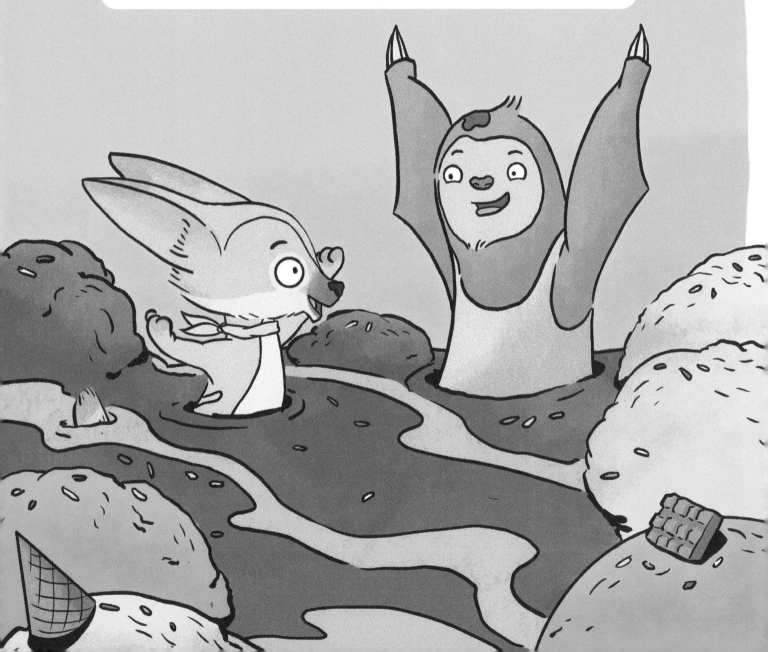

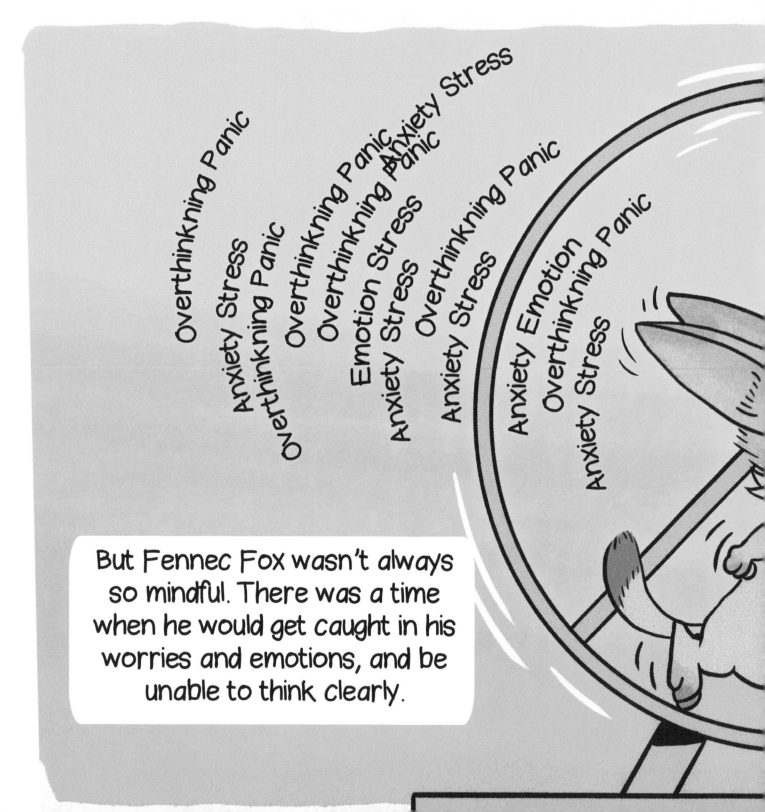

But Fennec Fox wasn't always so mindful. There was a time when he would get caught in his worries and emotions, and be unable to think clearly.

This was a very unhappy time for Fennec Fox.

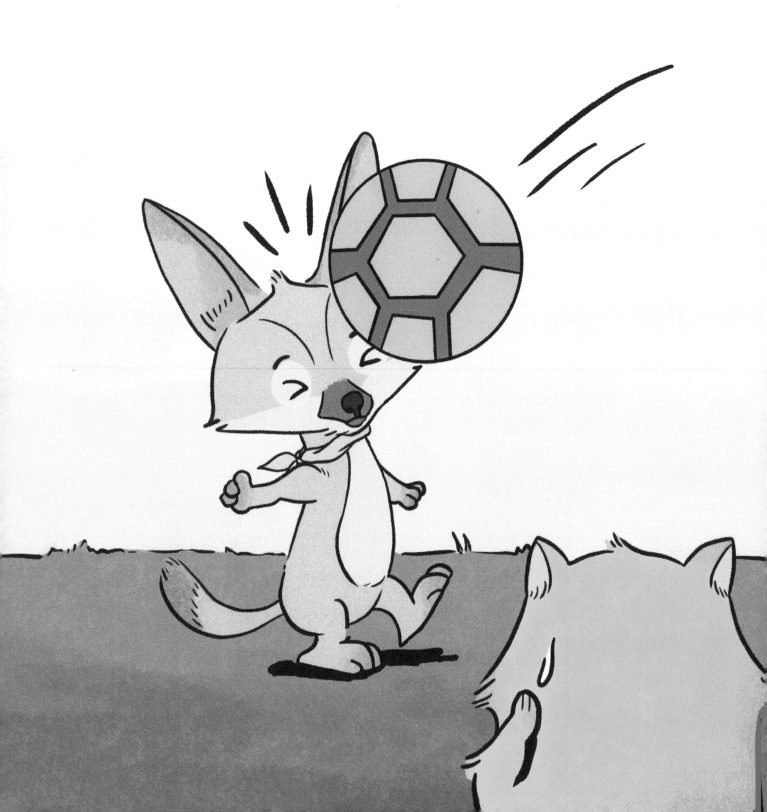

For example, Fennec Fox was afraid of trying new things like soccer out of fear that he would be bad, and his friends would think he was stupid.

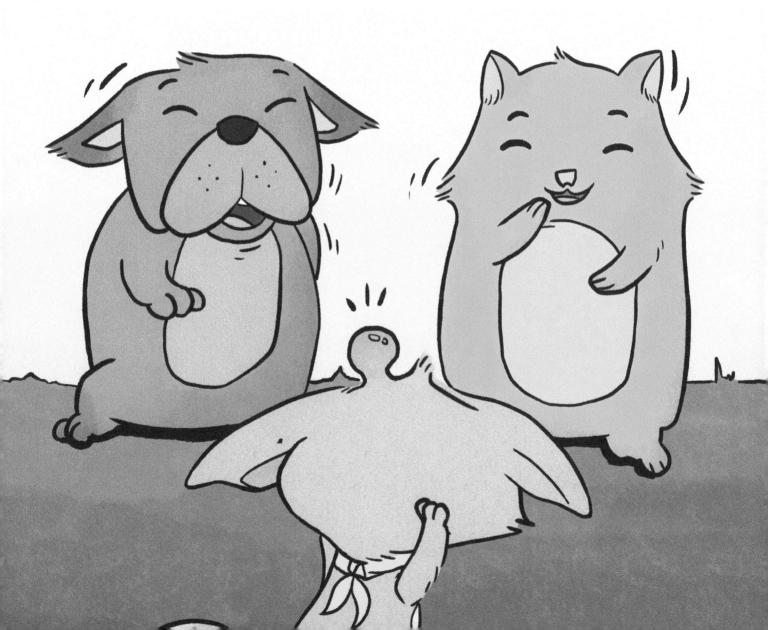

Once, someone cut in front of Fennec Fox at the lunch line and it made him so angry that he started screaming.

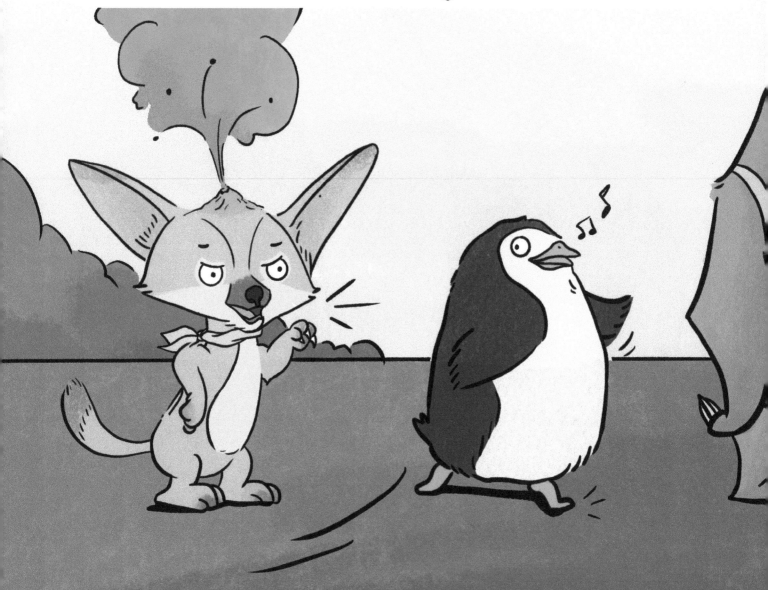

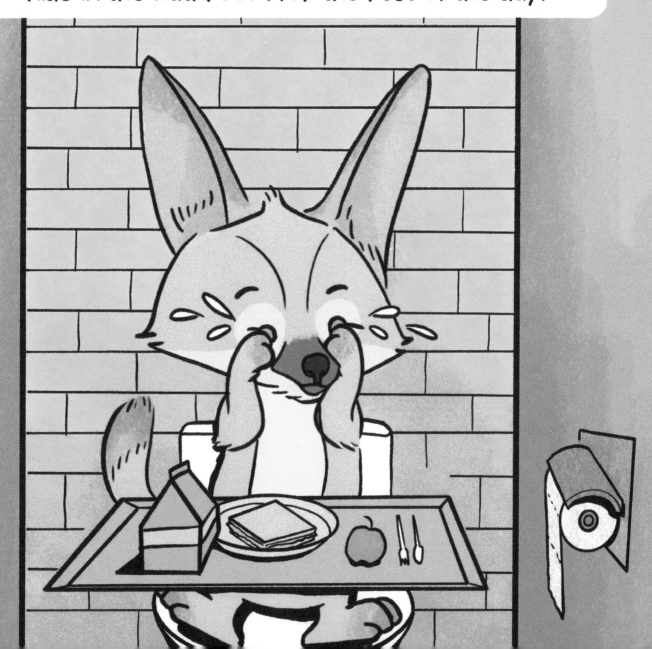

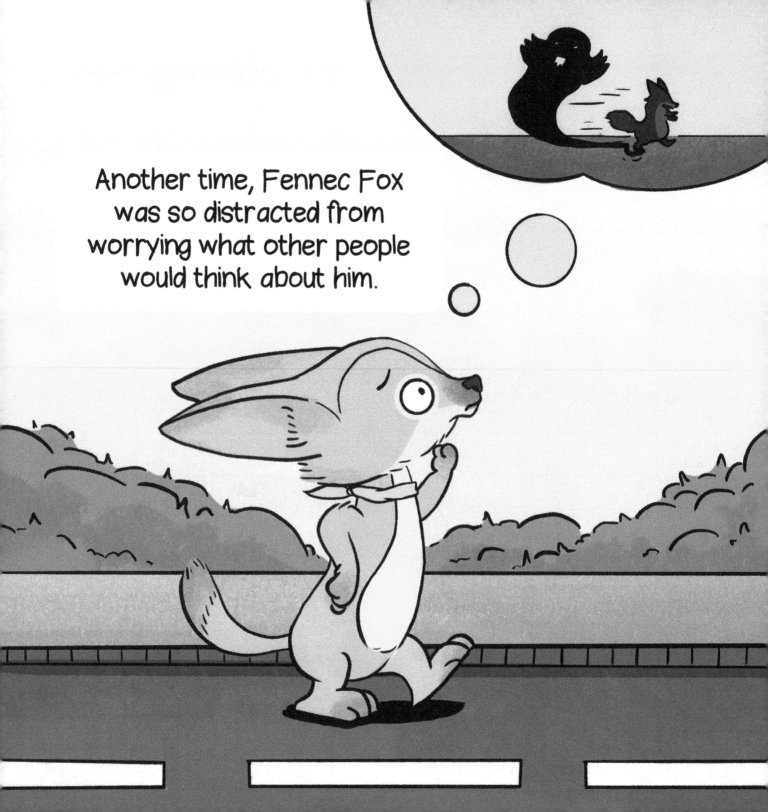

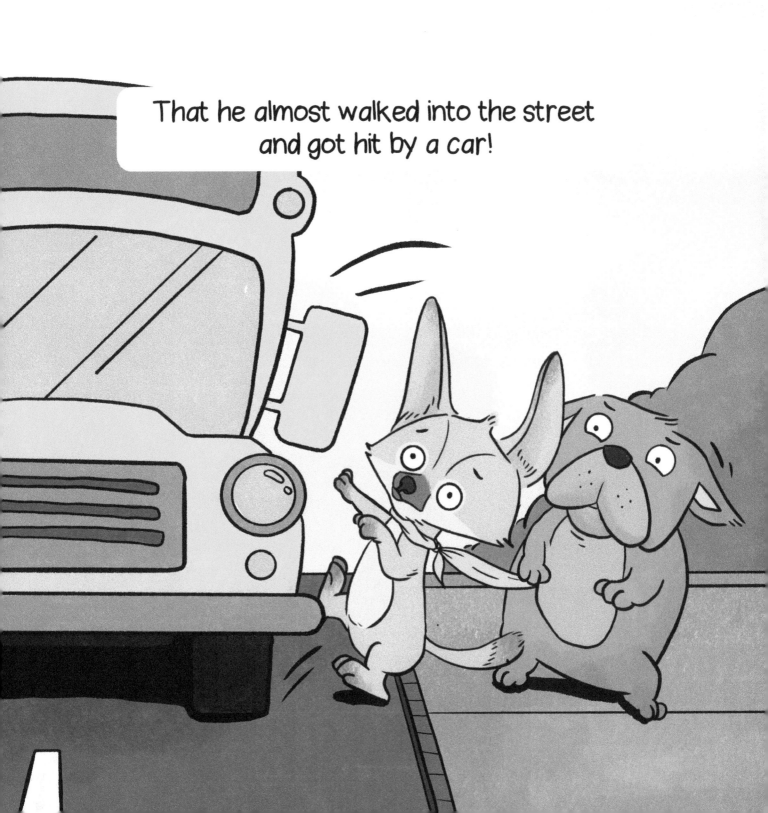

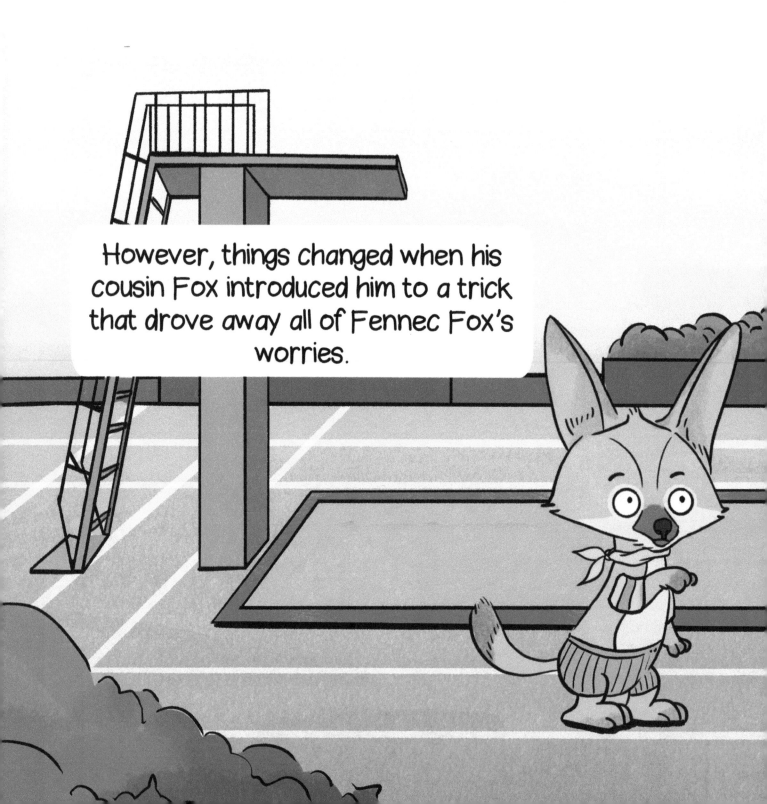

However, things changed when his cousin Fox introduced him to a trick that drove away all of Fennec Fox's worries.

Fox asked Fennec Fox to meet him
at the local pool.

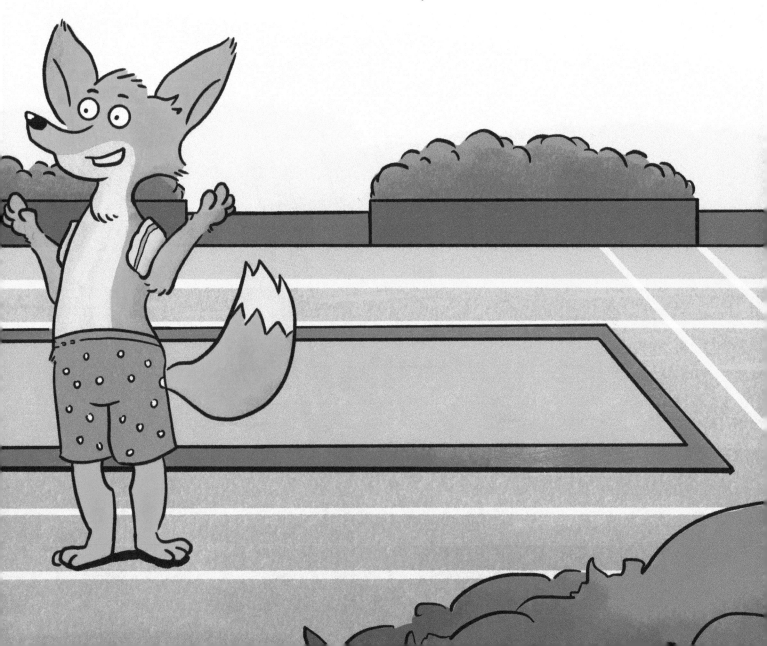

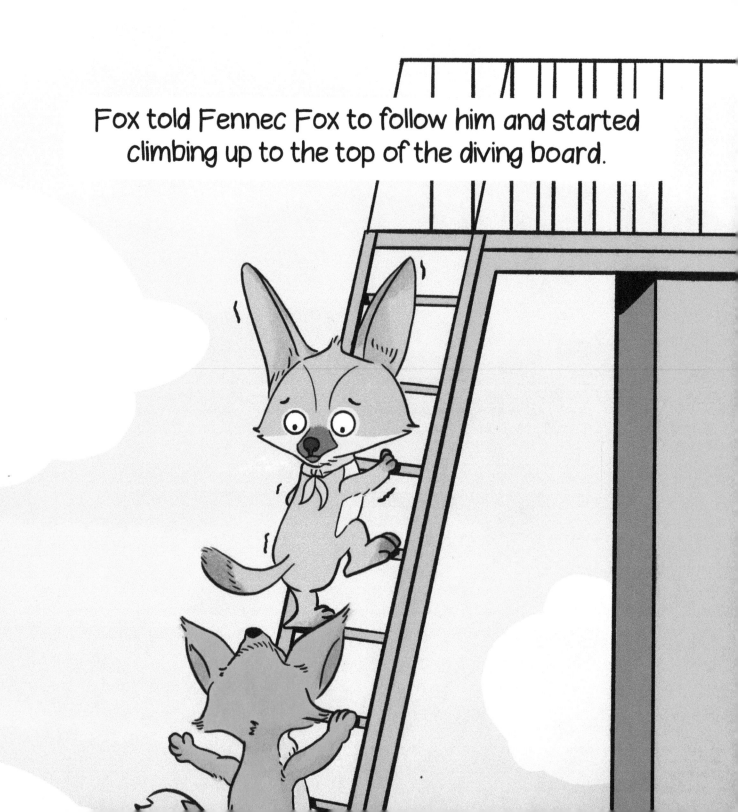

Fox told Fennec Fox to follow him and started climbing up to the top of the diving board.

Fennec Fox was not good with heights. In fact, he was very scared of them, and he didn't like deep water either!

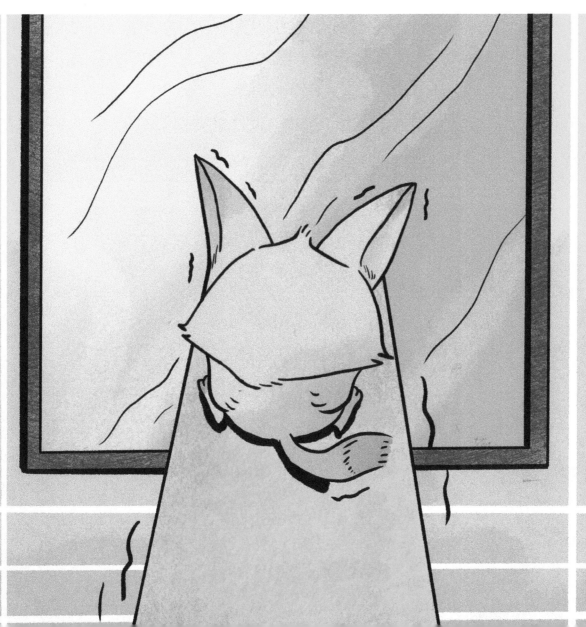

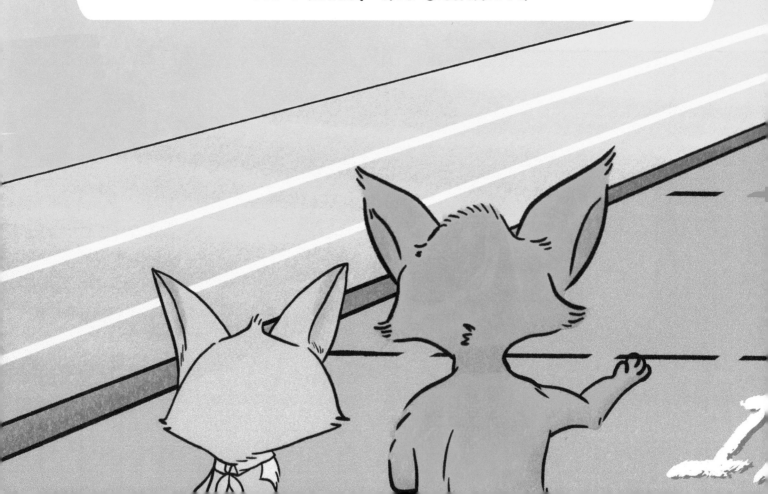

Fox said, "Whenever you feel yourself becoming overwhelmed by something negative, try using the 4-4-4-4 rule. That's easy to remember, right? This will keep you mindful, which means that you won't be taken away by your emotions or thoughts, and you can be in control and calm no matter the situation."

"This trick is about breathing! Inhale for 4 seconds, hold it for 4 seconds, and then exhale for 4 seconds. Then do this 4 times."

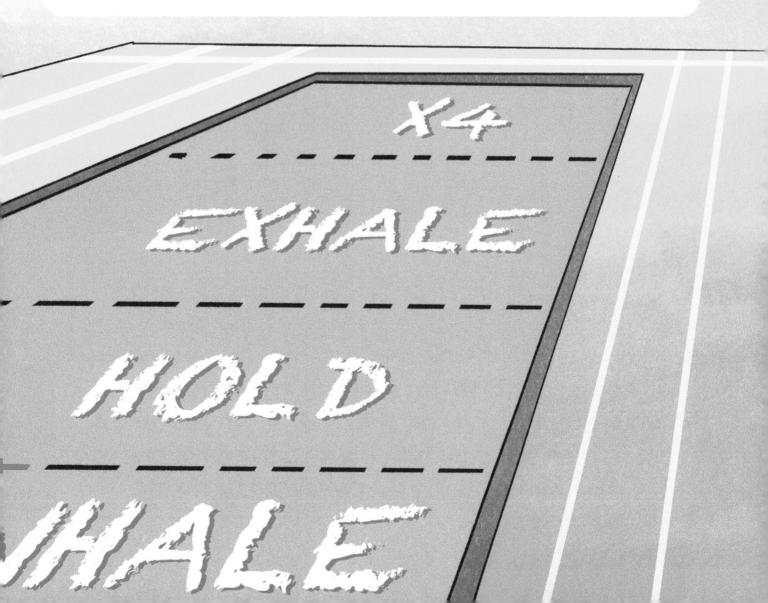

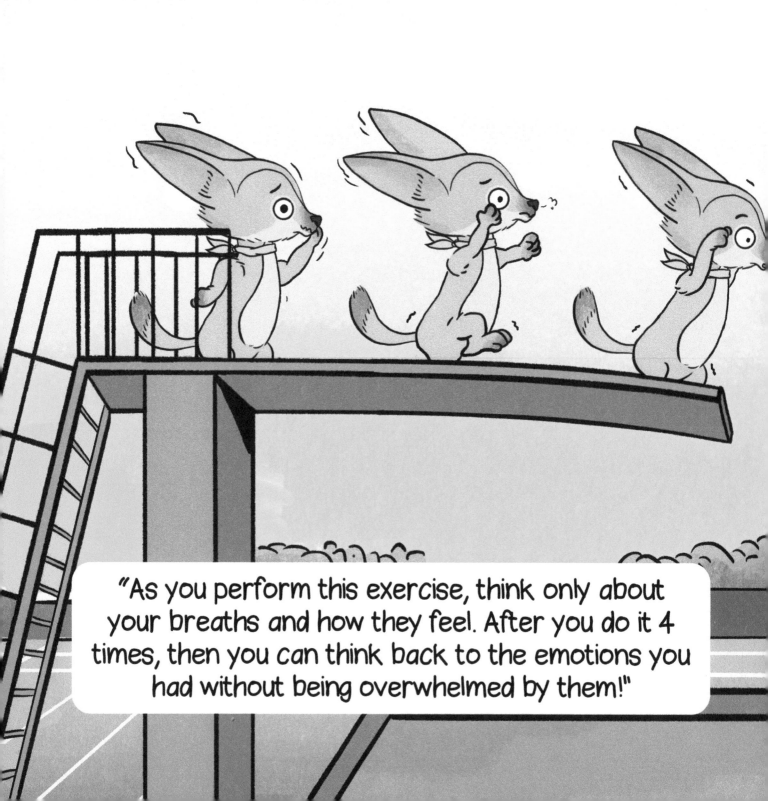

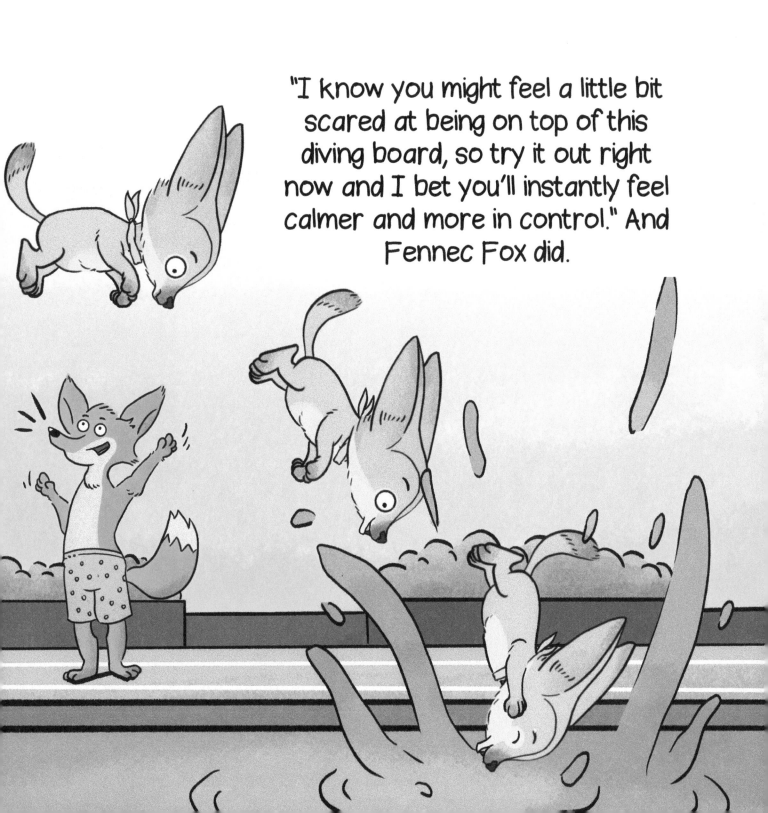

Fennec Fox was amazed. He felt like he had a new superpower! The next day at school, someone cut in front of him in the lunch line again!
How dare they!

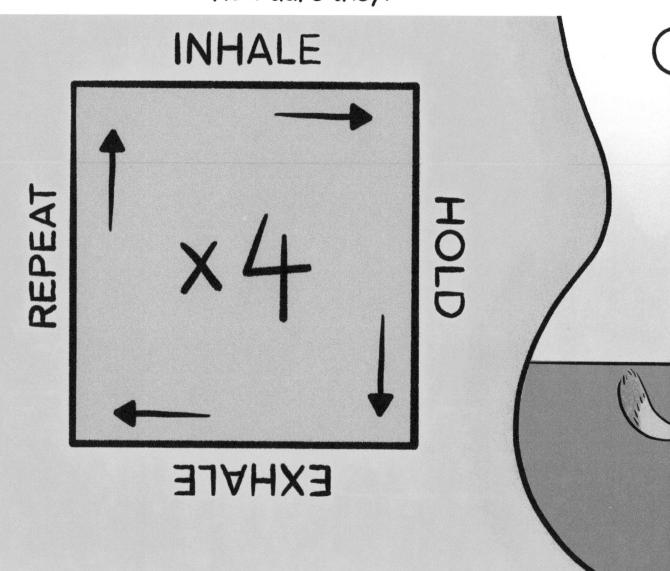

Fennec Fox almost blew up, but he tried the 4-4-4-4 rule and breathed until he could mindful.

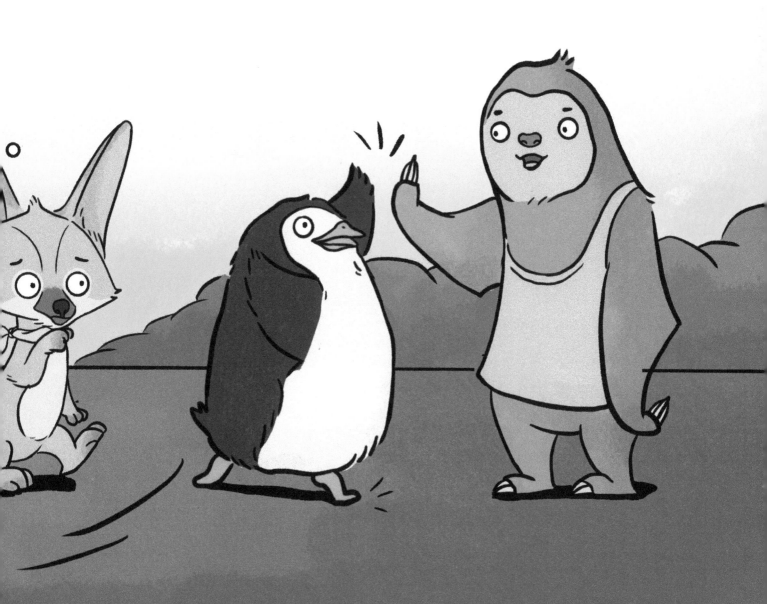

He was able to think about his emotions instead of being controlled by them. Success was his!

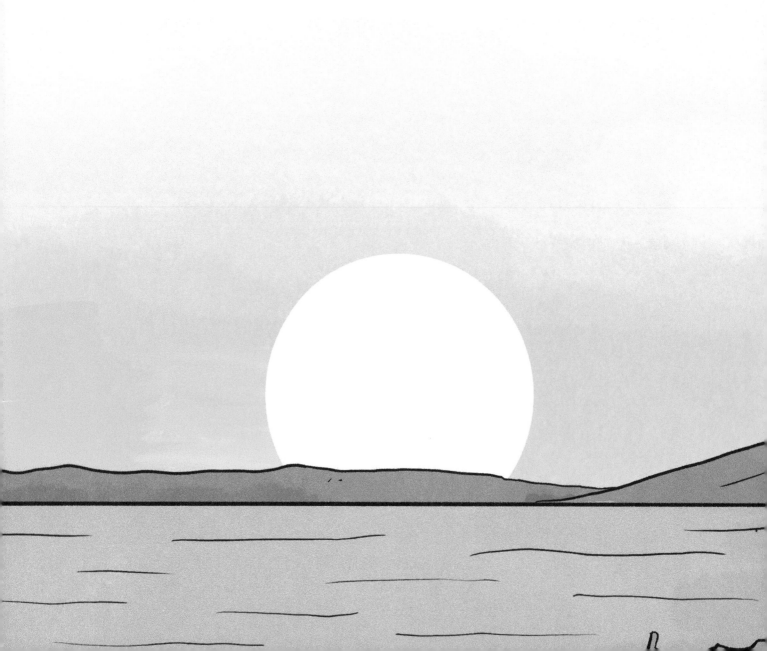

From that time onward, he used the 4-4-4-4 rule every time his brain felt too noisy, and he was being overwhelmed.

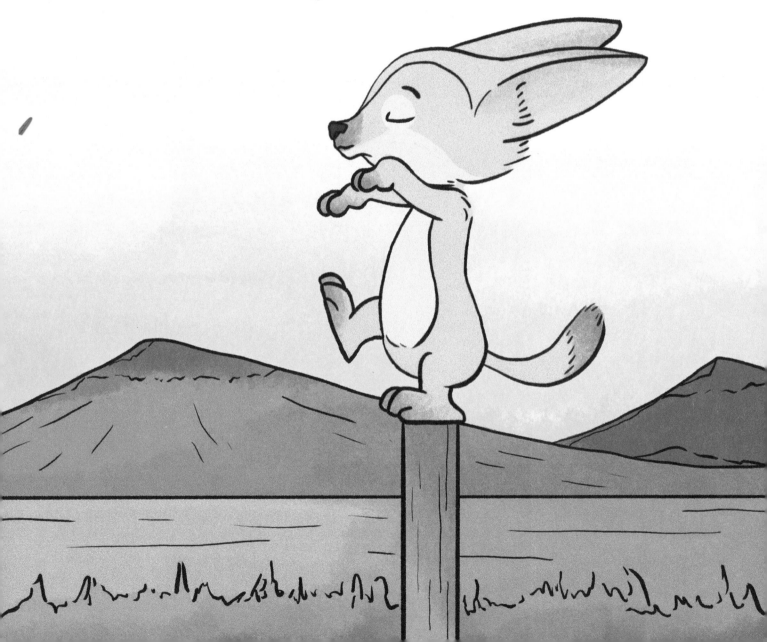

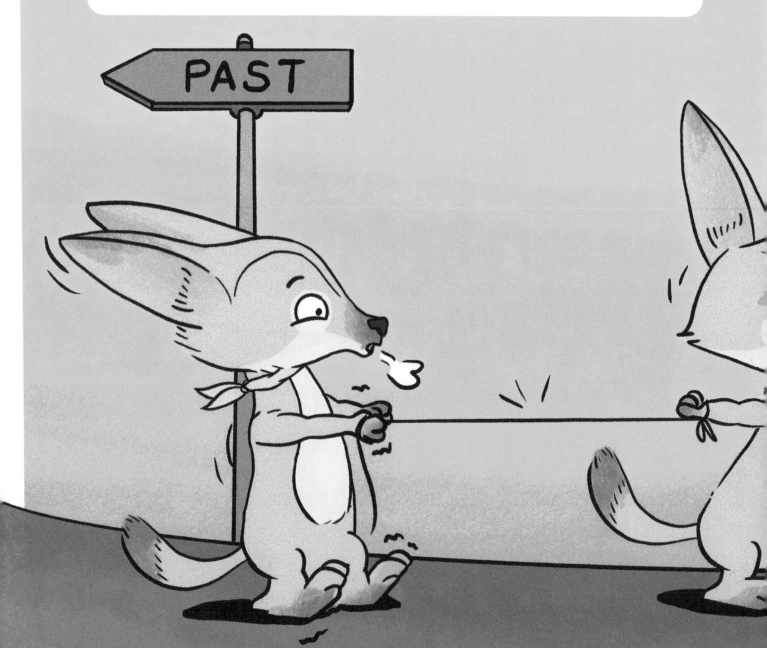

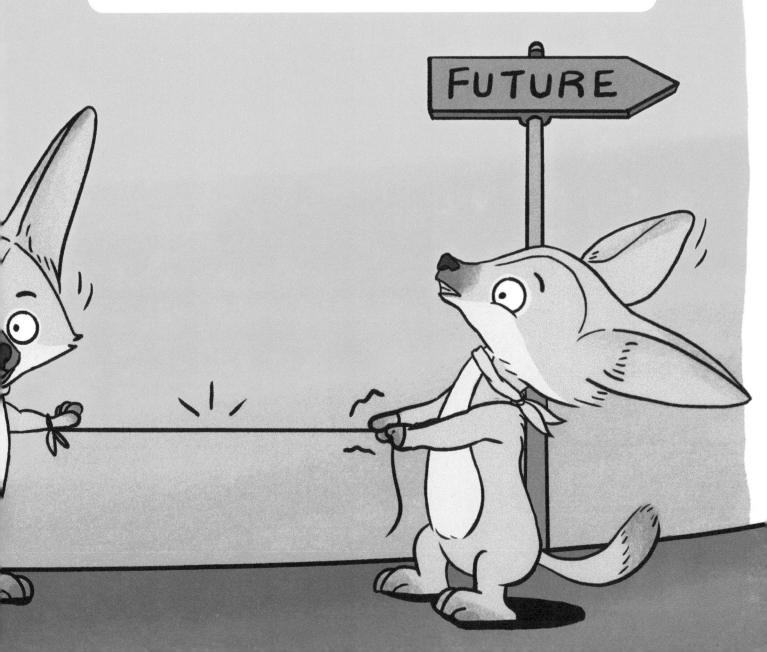

He realized how simple it was to be mindful. Emotions and distracting thoughts are powerful, but so was he!

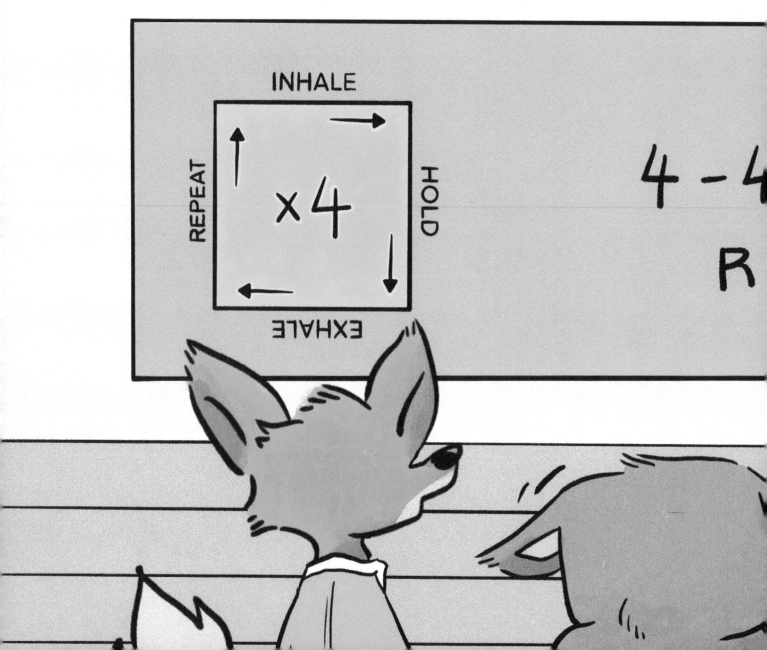

So many of Fennec Fox's problems could be solved by just taking deep breaths for a few minutes. Anyone can do it. The 4-4-4-4 rule can help you too to be mindful and in complete control.

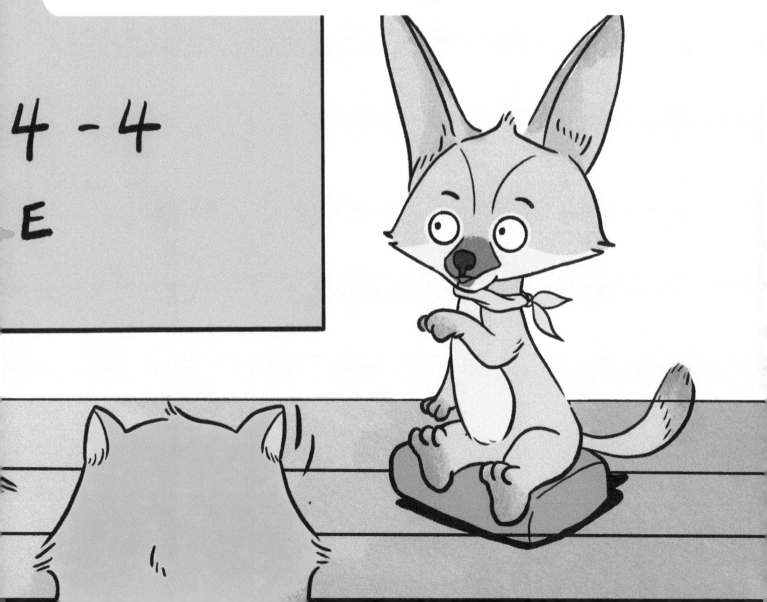

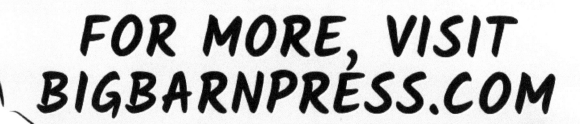

FOR MORE, VISIT
BIGBARNPRESS.COM

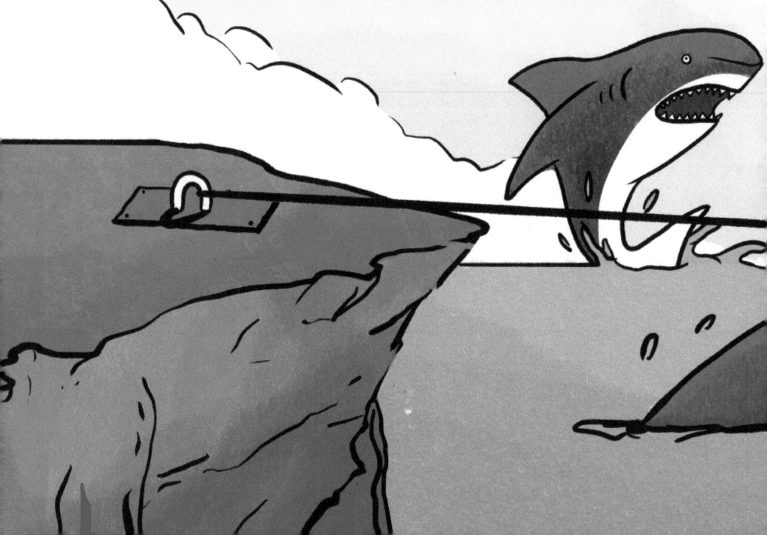

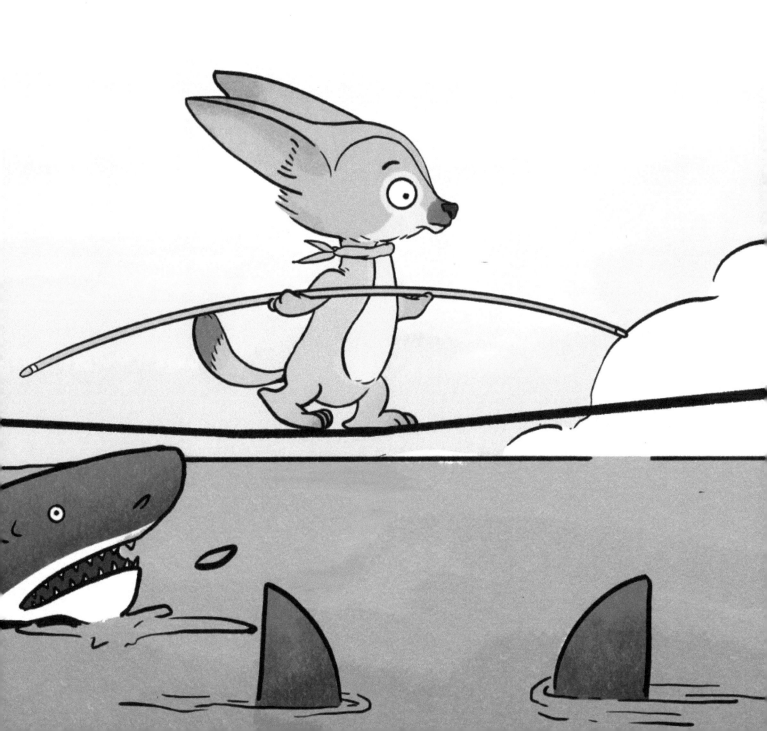

CPSIA information can be obtained
at www.ICGtesting.com
Printed in the USA
LVHW020724131220
674007LV00003B/96